Stomach Ulcer

Treatment, Home Remedies, Recipes

Table of Contents

Introduction

The stomach is a sensitive organ of the digestive system where the food eaten runs down the esophagus and is broken down further into smaller pieces before the small intestine can absorb the nutrients from the food. Various enzymes and acid are produced by the stomach digesting the food into simpler substances. A mucous layer protects the inner wall of the stomach from the enzymes and the acid.

The ulcers, or you can also call it "hell in the stomach", are caused due to the imbalance between the various factors that shields the stomach lining and the digestive juices of the stomach. The most alarming symptom of the stomach ulcer includes bleeding and rarely this may even erode the wall of the stomach! The bacterium Helicobacter pylorus is the main culprit behind this deadly disease. Treatment for this condition often includes medications like antibiotics to eradicate the infection or suppressors to limit the stomach acid generation. In worst cases, patients also need surgeries. Nowadays, stomach ulcer has become such an alarming issue that more and more people of all age groups are seen to suffer from the complications related to this condition. Necessary precautions and actions along with some few lifestyle changes need to be taken in order to lead a healthy life.

Chapter 1- Know about Stomach Ulcer

History of Stomach Ulcer in Brief

There is an interesting and a unique history behind the suspected causes of ulcers. Earlier in the 1880s, doctors used to treat stomach ulcers by performing surgeries that involved cutting off the stomach bottom reattached it to the intestines. However, many patients were not completely cured and some even severely bled causing them to die. Some patients could get cured through surgery, but around 25% of the stomach ulcer patients could never fully heal from the wound, became seriously ill and totally lost their appetite to eat food.

For several decades, stomach ulcers were related to high-stress lifestyle, also known as "psychosomatic". Eventually, high rates of ulcers were seen among hard-working businessmen who used to smoke plenty of cigarettes per day and used to get insufficient amount of sleep. These ulcers were further confirmed to be stress-triggered through animal studies.

According to some researches, scientists discovered that when rats are placed into high-pressure situations, acid damage and ulcer are developed inside the digestive tracts of the rats. When the researchers fed the rats antacids, the animals producing high level of stomach acid gradually began to experience a reduction in stomach ulcer symptoms. From this event, a conclusion was drawn that ulcers are linked with chronic stress and a rise in the level of stomach acid. After this, the approaches of treating ulcer have taken a new turn forever.

During that time, researchers discovered a bacterium name "Helicobacter Pylori" which was present in almost every patient suffering from stomach ulcers. This was also seen to be a hereditary health condition and was related to other digestive disorders too like stomach cancer. Ulcers were treated, or were kept benign for some time, by administrating patients with medicines or antibiotic to eradicate H. pylori bacteria. However, using antibiotics to kill H. pylori bacteria can cause complications including resistance to antibiotics. So, instead of using antibiotics, ulcers are treated by administrating less risky acid-reducing medicines along with dietary and lifestyle changes. Even though antibiotics can resist H. pylori for a while but it cannot completely stop the bacteria from returning without other interventions.

According to the speculation of some researchers, by the beginning of the 20th century unfortunately all of the mankind was infected with this bacterium and could lead their whole lives without having a symptom at all. Doctors further discovered that the infection caused by H. pylori is more likely to trigger the ulcers. Since the bacteria cannot cause the ulcer pain alone, there must be something else too that made some patients particularly susceptible to the condition. Later, it became widely established that a person's lifestyle and hygiene can determine if the person will be affected by this bacteria or suffer from the symptoms at all. Apart from the amount of contaminated food and water intake, the chances of developing stomach ulcer also increases with the level of inflammation and stress a person goes through.

Understanding Your Gut and Digestion

Before you go through the discussion about the basic mechanism of stomach ulcer, you must know how your gut and digestive system work.

The food that you eat goes down the esophagus, the food pipe, of the stomach. The stomach then generates acid that helps in digestion of the food, although not necessary. After the acid gets amalgamated with the food, the food then enters into the duodenum which is the first part of the small intestine. This food is then gets mixed with digestive chemicals called enzymes inside the duodenum and the rest of the small intestine. These enzymes are secreted from the inner lining of the intestine and the pancreas. The enzymes then digest, or break down, the food that is absorbed into the body.

Basic Mechanism of Stomach Ulcer

A stomach ulcer causes erosion in the gastrointestinal tract of a person. An ulcer is also known as a 'Peptic ulcer'. Duodenal ulcer is the most commonly seen ulcer among patients. This happens within the first end of a person's small intestine, just past their stomach. Gastric ulcer is the type of ulcer that is formed in the patient's stomach. Duodenal ulcer is mostly benign whereas stomach ulcer may become malignant in some cases. Ulcers are neither contagious nor cancerous, so don't lose hope if you are suffering from this disease. It can be treated. Millions of Americans suffer from this disease per year. The size of an ulcer ranges from $1/8^{th}$ to $3/4^{th}$ of an inch.

Stomach ulcers are common in mastocytosis, and can act as a symptom of other diseases and health conditions. A person may experience iron deficiency anemia if he or she bleeds due to stomach ulcers. Stomach ulcer may also develop in children. Around 20 million Americans suffer from at least 1 stomach ulcer in their lifetime. More than 40,000 Americans have to go through surgeries per year due to persistent complications and symptoms of stomach ulcers. On the other hand, around 6000 Americans die due to complications related to stomach ulcer each year.

As stated earlier, the stomach is a sack of muscle that combines and breaks down the consumed food with hydrochloric acid and the enzyme pepsin. When the stomach lining or the duodenum of patient experiences damage, the acid and the enzyme works on the stomach lining in the same way as these would do with the food eaten. This erodes the lining as lining and would digest it instead of food. Too much secretion of the acid and the pepsin would destroy a person's stomach lining resulting in an ulcer. Other reasons may also cause this damage, turning the patient's stomach more vulnerable to normal levels of gastric acid.

Ulcer patients who ignore the symptoms or remain untreated can experience severe bleeding. In bleeding ulcers, the wound enters into the patient's blood vessels making the blood to seep into the digestive tract. Patients may also suffer from perforated ulcer that erodes a hole in the stomach wall or the duodenum, causing bacteria and the partially digested food entering into the hole and resulting in inflammation. Untreated patients are also likely to experience a constriction or narrowing of their intestinal opening that resists food from going out of their stomach and entering into small intestine.

Some Terms Explained

- **Peptic inflammation** – This is the inflammation caused that is caused by stomach acid. The inflammation may occur in the stomach particularly in the first region of the small intestine (or, the duodenum) or in the esophagus (the lower gullet). This happens as the stomach acid flows in with the swallowed food and the acid splashes up resulting in "reflux esophagus".
- **Peptic ulcer** – This condition is caused by stomach acid. Ulcers occur when the gut lining are destroyed and the essential tissue remains exposed. An ulcer looks like a small red hole on the inner lining of the gut.

- **Stomach ulcer** – It is a type of peptic ulcer and is also known as gastric ulcer. However, the most common type of peptic ulcer is the duodenum ulcer.

Stomach ulcers are common. According to the American Gastroenterological Association, an estimated 4 million Americans have peptic ulcer disease, which includes duodenal ulcers.

Did You Know?

- Statistics show that around 500,000 new cases of peptic ulcers have been known to get reported per year in the U.S alone. At any given time of the year around 5 million citizens become infected. Moreover, 1 in 10 adults is more likely to experience painful ulcers at some point.
- Abdominal pains and burning sensations are the most common symptoms of stomach ulcer. The bleeding takes place when the patient goes to the bathroom or when he or she vomits. Other symptoms include nausea, darker stools, appetite loss, risk of organ lining perforation, reduction in body weight, acid reflux, dehydration, sleep-deprived due to intolerable pain, weakness, fatigue, heartburn, feeling gassy, and other digestive complaints.

- High percentage of ulcer cases (around 90%) can be cured without going through any surgery or heavy doses of medicines.
- Men mostly develop duodenum ulcers than other the types. On the other hand, women are more likely to develop stomach ulcers and some duodenum ulcers. Generally, women develop ulcers more than men, especially over the age of 70, and have to take medicines and drugs regularly. The most vulnerable age range of developing ulcers is 55 to 65 years.
- Stomach ulcer can be naturally treated by restricting the use of NSAID pain killers, boosting immunity, controlling stress level and inflammation and by eating more nutrient-rich diet and low-processed food.

Chapter 2 –Stomach Ulcer: Causes & Symptoms

If you have read the above literature, then you know all about the 'what(s)' of stomach ulcer. This chapter is a bit lengthy but is worth reading as it will describe the causes, symptoms, and other vital information regarding stomach ulcer.

What Causes Stomach Ulcers?

Generally, stomach produces corrosive acid to kill bacteria, germs and to digest food. A natural mucous barrier is produced by some cells on the inner lining of stomach and the first region of small intestine due to the corrosiveness of the stomach acid. The mucous layer protects the lining of the duodenum and the stomach. Typically, your body maintains a balance between the amount of acid secretion and the defense barrier. Whenever the system becomes imbalanced, ulcer develops, and the acid can harm the lining of duodenum and the stomach. Some causes that result in stomach ulcer are:

❖ **Infection with Helicobacter pylori (H. pylori)**

In about 8 out of 10 cases of stomach ulcer, the main culprit behind is the H. pylori. In UK, more than 1/4th of the population become infected with the H. pylori bacteria at some point of their lives.

Once you are infected, the bacteria stay in your body throughout your whole life, unless you are treated. Many victims experience no problem at all and the bacteria live harmlessly inside the lining of the duodenum and the stomach. Unfortunately, some victims experience inflammation in the stomach or duodenum lining and disrupt the defense mucous barrier and also increase the amount of acid production that eventually causes ulcers and inflammation.

❖ **Anti-inflammatory medicines**

Anti-inflammatory medicines are sometimes known as non-steroidal anti-inflammatory drugs (NSAIDs). There are many kinds and brands of NSAIDs medicines, such as ibuprofen, diclofenac, aspirin and many more. A lot of people take anti-inflammatory medicine for muscle pain, arthritis etc. People often take aspirin to protect against formation of blood clots. These drugs, however, affect the mucous barrier of stomach and cause an ulcer by the acid. About 2 out of 10 stomach ulcer cases are triggered by anti-inflammatory drugs.

❖ **Lifestyle factors**

People used to think that certain lifestyle factors may cause stomach ulcers. The factors include stress, alcohol, smoking and spicy foods. Even though there isn't many evidence that these factors are the villain but these can make things worse.

❖ Other factors and causes

Other causes and factors can be seen rarely. For instances, stomach ulcer can be caused by some viral infections. In addition to other issues of your gut, stomach ulcer may also occur due to Crohn's disease. At first, stomach cancer may appear similar to an ulcer. Stomach cancer is not a common case and may need not to be considered if you are diagnosed with stomach ulcer. There are some behaviors and factors that can increase the risk of developing stomach ulcers:

- Frequent steroids intake (e.g. treating asthma)
- Smoking
- Excessive drinking of alcohol
- Hypercalcemia (excess generation of calcium)
- Being over 50 years old
- Family medical history of developing stomach ulcer
- Imbalance diet, irregularity or skipped meals
- Stress
- Intake of corticosteroids or non-steroidal anti-inflammatory drugs
- Zollinger-Ellison syndrome
- Type O blood
- Rheumatic arthritis, emphysema, liver disease or other chronic diseases

Signs and Symptoms of Stomach Ulcer

Burning sensation and a gnawing feeling inside the stomach are the major symptoms of having an ulcer. The symptoms may last from 30 minutes to several hours, depending on the seriousness of the situation. People often associate the pain, caused due to ulcer, with indigestion, heartburn or hunger. Some unfortunates experience the pain immediately after eating, while others do not even feel anything for hours. Ulcer patients may experience extreme pain that wake them up at night. There are also some patients who feel this pain for weeks and then this pain goes away completely for next couple of weeks. The nerves surrounding a stomach ulcer get harmed by the ulcer and can cause pain, making the nerves agitated. Stomach ulcer patients may also suffer from hemorrhages as the major blood vessels become eroded or the patients' stomach and intestinal wall get torn. The results are may be caused due to peritonitis or an obstruction of the patient's gastrointestinal tract. This happens because of spasm or swelling in the region of the person's ulcer.

As stated earlier, stomach burning or gnawing pain in the middle of the tummy (abdomen) is the most common sign of having a stomach ulcer.

Stomach ulcer doesn't cause pain always and can only be noticed when you experience a complication regarding stomach ulcer, like bleeding due to ulcer. Some patients also experience other signs and symptoms like heartburn, indigestion of feel sickness.

- **Tummy pain**

The stomach pain caused by the ulcer starts from the centre of the tummy and reach up to the neck, then it travels down the belly button or your back. The pain can sustain from a few hours to few hours, or often begins after some hours of eating. Patients may also wake up in the night due to pain. The pain can be relieved temporarily by taking antacids or other medicines for indigestion, but it will return if the ulcers are left untreated.

- **Other symptoms**

There are other signs that indicate you are suffering from stomach ulcer, and these include loss of appetite, heartburn, indigestion, weight loss and feeling sick. Some patients even feel bloated or burp after eating fatty meals.

When to Seek Medical Advice

In case you feel the symptoms of stomach ulcers persistently, then you should pay a visit to a GP or a nearby hospital.

You must not delay if you see the following symptoms:

- **Vomiting blood** – the blood may look like dark brown or bright red with grainy texture, similar to coffee powder
- Passing stools that have sticky and dark appearance
- Black or dark stool due to bleeding
- A sharp, sudden pain in the tummy that increases and become worse eventually

Patients may experience other symptoms or serious complications, such as severe internal bleeding. Whatever the signs or symptoms are, you must never delay and should immediately rush to the doctor before it becomes too late.

How Serious is an Ulcer?

Most of the time ulcers heal on their own, however, you must never overlook the warming symptoms. If left untreated as then ulcers may lead to detrimental health issues, like:

- **Internal bleeding**

The most common complication of stomach ulcer is internal bleeding. This can take place when an ulcer forms at the location of blood vessels. The bleeding can be:

- **Severe and rapid bleeding** – make you vomit blood release stools that are sticky, black and look like tar.

- **Long-term, slow bleeding eventually causing anemia -** you will experience breathlessness, fatigue, noticeable heart palpitations and have pale skin.

The cause of the bleeding will be diagnosed by performing an **endoscopy**. Necessary treatments will be given during the process to stop further bleeding. Specialized procedures are sometimes performed while doing X-ray in order to stop bleeding from ulcers, even though surgery can occasionally be needed to fix the harmed blood vessels. In this case, **blood transfusions** may also be required to replace the lost blood.

- **Perforation**

Perforation is term used to describe the splitting of the stomach lining caused by stomach ulcers. This is a rare complication and can proof to be very serious since it allows the bacteria residing in your stomach to come out and infect the lining of your peritoneum (abdomen). This condition is also known as **peritonitis**. Victims suffering from this condition can have their infections rapidly spread into their bloodstreams (sepsis) prior to spreading in other organs. If left untreated, this can be detrimental to health since this can cause multiple organ damage.

The most common peritonitis is a sharp, sudden pain in the abdomen that gets worse gradually. In case you experience this type of pain, you must contact your doctor immediately.

If you cannot do this, call your local out-of-hours service such as NHS 111. Patients suffering from this medical emergency needs to be admitted in the hospital and in some cases, they may need surgeries.

- **Gastric outlet obstruction**

There are many cases where patients having a swollen or an inflamed, scarred stomach ulcer may experience hindrance in the flow of food through their digestive system. This condition is also called **gastric outlet obstruction** and the symptoms are:

- Persistently feeling fullness or bloated
- Feeling heavy or full after consuming less food than usual
- Vomit repeatedly and puking out large amount of undigested food chunks
- Unnatural weight loss

The obstruction can be confirmed by performing endoscopy. If inflammation is the main reason behind the obstruction, you need to use proton pump inhibitors (PPIs) or H2-receptor antagonists in order to decrease levels of stomach ulcer until the inflammation goes down. If scar tissues cause these obstructions, then you may need surgery to treat it. However, sometimes it can also be treated by passing a tiny balloon or a blob through the endoscopy and simultaneously inflating it to make the site of the obstructions wider.

Who is More Likely to Develop Ulcers?

Various parts of the GI tract can develop ulcers, like in stomach, duodenum and the esophagus. However, it is interesting to know from several researches that more often men suffer from duodenal ulcers, particularly in the small intestines, compared to other types of ulcers. Contrary to common belief, women are like to develop more stomach ulcers and less duodenal ulcers than men.

In general cases, women tend to suffer from ulcers more than men, especially if their age is 70 years or more and regularly use over–the-counter medications and drugs. The most vulnerable age to get ulcers is from 55 to 65 years. The immunity system of people tends to become weaker and have increasing risk of developing inflammation as they grow older. This raises the chance of getting more H. pylori infections that harms the stomach lining and can cause bleeding ulcers. According to some studies, H. pylori are 60 percent more abundant among older people with duodenal and gastric ulcers than others. Several doctors consider stomach ulcers as peptic ulcers. Ulcers are also known as:

- **Duodenal ulcers** – The duodenum is the nearest region of the small intestine that has length of about 10 inches and plays a vital role in digesting the food by holding the bile. The pancreatic duct and the bile duct both empty their contents into the duodenum. Therefore, this can be dilated or obstructed when the amount of bile production alters in response to other activities in the body.
- **Esophageal ulcers** – This is a type of peptic ulcer that is formed right above the stomach in the esophagus. The esophagus if the long tube that carries the food you eat from your mouth down to organs of the digestive system.
- **Bleeding ulcers** – Untreated ulcers can start bleeding anytime and can arouse other complications. Bleeding ulcers are the most dangerous of all other types. When there is a ruptured blood vessel in your small intestine or stomach, internal bleeding can also take part in ulcers.
- **Gastric ulcers** – The amount of hyperacidity of the gastric juices increases in some ulcer patients which alters the effects of stomach acid on the GI tract lining. Generally, gastric ulcers are actually small openings in the stomach wall that can cause formation of stomach ulcers.

You are more prone to develop ulcers when you:

- Intake NSAIDs like ibuprofen, naproxen or aspirin
- Become infected with H. pylori bacteria

- Have medical history of ulcers in the family
- Suffer from illness like kidney, lung, or liver disease
- Regularly drink alcohol
- Age of 50 or above

Chapter 3 – Be Deterrent, Analyse and Treat It Well

Before jumping into any conclusion, the first and foremost task must be to properly diagnose the main reason or underlying health issue that is causing all the signs and symptoms of low blood pressure. In this case, your doctor will prescribe you some tests or procedures to identify the main culprit behind. Only after this, proper treatment and medical assistance can be availed. At the end of this chapter, some tips are given on how to prevent low blood pressure and complications related to it.

Diagnosis

For the sake of detecting an ulcer, your doctor will take your medical history from you and will carry out a physical exam. Then you will have to go through some diagnostic tests, like:

- **Laboratory tests for H. pylori.** You doctor may prescribe you to do some tests to find out if the H. pylori bacteria are present inside your body. The H. pylori can be traced by doing a stool, blood or breath test. The most accurate test is the breath tests. Generally, blood tests are not accurate and routine use should be avoided.

H. pylori can be traced via stool, breath or blood tests. The most accurate test is the breath test while blood tests are generally not accurate and regular use should be avoided. For breath test, you have to eat or drink something that is radioactive carbon. The H. pylori bacteria breaks down this in your stomach and after a while you blow into a bag. The bag is sealed with your breath sample. If you are infected, then your breath sample with have traces of radioactive carbon as carbon dioxide. You must inform your doctor if you have taken antacid before doing the test for H. pylori. You need to discontinue the medicine for a while depending on the type of test you have to do.

- **Endoscopy.** You doctor may look for a scope to test your upper digestive system and this process is called endoscopy. During the procedure, the doctors pass a hollow tube with a lens attached (endoscope) down the throat and towards the esophagus, stomach and small intestine. By doing the endoscope, the doctors search for ulcers. If an ulcer is detected, then a small tissue portion (biopsy) will be removed for testing in the lab. The biopsy can also detect H. pylori bacteria inside the stomach wall. If you are older, experience bleeding, appetite loss, difficulty in eating and swallowing, or recently notice unusual weight loss, then you have to do endoscopy.

If the report shows a stomach ulcer, then you will have to do a follow-up endoscopy after treatment to see if your ulcer has healed, even if the symptoms go away.

- **Upper gastrointestinal series.** This is often known as barium swallow. This series of X-rays of the upper digestive system produces images of the esophagus, small intestine and the stomach. Before starting the test, you will be given white barium liquid to swallow to coat your digestive tract and makes the ulcers more noticeable.

- **Biopsy.** A small sample of tissue is taken while doing endoscopy and is examined in the lab. This test must always be done if the doctors find a gastric ulcer.

- **C14 breathe test.** This test for the presence of H. pylori. This bacterium can turn urea into carbon dioxide. In this test, you will have to swallow C14 (a radioactive carbon) and examine the exhaled air from the lungs. For pregnant women and children, a non-radioactive test can be done.

Treatment of Stomach Ulcer

If you are diagnosed with an ulcer, the treatment for you will depend on the cause of it. Having proper treatment, many ulcers are cured in about a couple of months.

If you are suffering from stomach ulcer caused by H. pylori bacteria infection, then you will be recommended to take a course of antibiotics and a medicine called proton pump inhibitor (PPI). This is advised if the cause of ulcer is a combination of H. pylori bacteria and non-steroidal anti-inflammatory drugs (NSAIDs). Patients of stomach ulcer caused by taking NSAIDs are advised to take PPI medicines. Your doctor will review your use of NSAIDs and may also recommend you an alternative painkiller. Occasionally, an alternative medicine, called H2-receptor antagonist, is used instead of PPIs. Sometimes you may be prescribed additional antacids to relieve you from suffering of the signs in short term. Your doctor will check whether the ulcer is healed by repeating the gastroscopy after 4 to 6 weeks. You need not to make any special lifestyle changes while undergoing the treatment, but try to avoid consuming alcohol, spicy foods, avoid stress and smoking to lessen the symptoms when the ulcer heals.

❖ **Antibiotics**

In case you are infected with H. pylori bacteria, doctors will prescribe you a course of antibiotics for 2 to 3 weeks and you will need to be taken 2 times a day for 1 week. The most commonly used antibiotics are amoxicillin, metronidazole and clarithromycin.

These medicines have mild side-effects like diarrhea, metallic taste in the mouth and feeling sick. After completing the course of your antibiotic, you will be tested again minimum after 4 weeks to see if you are cured and the bacteria are eradicated from your stomach completely. There are also other therapies to wipe out the bacteria from your body and you can try those if your doctor suggests.

❖ Proton Pump Inhibitors (PPIs)

As the stomach heals naturally, PPI prevents further damage to the ulcer by limiting the amount of acid produced by the stomach. Usually, these are advised to take for 4 to 8 weeks. The most common PPIs used to treat stomach ulcers include lansoprazole, pantoprazole and omeprazole. These medicines have mild side-effects, like dizziness, headaches, feeling sick, rashes, diarrhea, tummy or abdominal pain or constipation. These will go away as soon as the treatment is done.

❖ H2-receptor antagonists

Just like the PPIs, H2-receptor antagonists also perform by lessening the acid production by the stomach. The most widely used H2-receptor in treating stomach ulcer is ranitidine. They usually don't have any side-effect, although they may induce headaches, rashes, diarrhea, tiredness or dizziness.

❖ **Antacids and alginates**

Several hours may take for the above mentioned treatments before they begin to act. In this case, your doctor may advise you to take additional antacid medicines to neutralize the stomach acid so that you'll get immediate relief, even though for short-time. Some antacids also contain alginate that generates a protective layer on the stomach lining. You can buy these medicines from over-the-counter pharmacies. The pharmacist can suggest you the suitable option for you. You should take antacids at bedtime or before meals, that is, when you experience complications or when you expect them. It is best to take alginates containing antacids after eating food. Minor side-effects can be noticed in both the medicines and they are feeling sick, diarrhea, stomach cramps, constipation or flatulence (wind).

❖ **Surgical treatment**

A complicated stomach ulcer will need surgeries in very rare cases. These types of ulcers continue to come back, bleed, don't heal easily, prevent food from going out of the stomach into the small intestine and break the small intestine or stomach lining. Surgery may need to take tissue from another region of intestines and sew it on the ulcer, remove the entire ulcer, seal the nerve supply to the stomach to decrease the stomach acid generation, and closing a bleeding artery.

Natural Treatment Plan of Stomach Ulcer

If you have a doubt that you might have developed stomach ulcer, immediately consult your doctor to rule out other reasons of pain. The doctor will at first take your and your family's medical history and do some physical tests, including blood test and might also do an X-ray to locate a possible stomach ulcer. The main aim of treating a stomach ulcer is to reduce the excruciating pain and inflammation in your GI tract, enhance your immunity system to combat against H. pylori bacteria, cure the complications and reduce the risk of reforming ulcers in the future.

1. Limit use of NSAIDs pain killers

Frequent users of NSAIDs (like Advil or ibuprofen) of any age group are more prone to suffer from stomach ulcers and heartburn compared to other people who don't use them much. These medicines are often prescribed by doctors to treat pain, swelling, fever and some people even take them regularly to get relief from arthritis/joint pain, PMS cramps, muscle tears, infections, colds, headaches and other chronic or reoccurring pains. The GI system gets damaged by these medicines by changing how stomach acids and digestive enzymes are secreted. Pain, fever and inflammation promoting chemicals are produced by 2 enzymes in your body.

NSAIDs reduce these enzymes and simultaneously decrease the production of chemicals that shields the stomach wall from getting damaged by stomach acid. If possible, either stop or limit the use of NSAIDs drugs or use alternative pain killers by consulting your doctor.

You might be wondering that taking antacids and acid-reducing drugs may cure ulcers. You might get temporary relief from a stomach ulcer by taking antacids but it will continue to return if the underlying cause remains untreated. You doctor my prescribe you antacids or other medicines to coat and protect the ulcer, but at the end of the day you'll want to control the symptoms naturally for a long time instead of becoming dependent on medicines.

2. Manage stress

Even though the theory of stress being the culprit behind causing stomach ulcer has not been fully proven, stress still plays a crucial role in the stomach ulcer development and this condition is still known as psychosomatic. Patients suffering from chronic stress, the risk of developing stomach ulcer increases. This happens because of the strong gut-brain connection with the digestive system. If your body experiences any perceived threat, then the normal process of digestion is hindered. That's why depressed or frustrated people complain about digestive problems more than other.

Patients with anxiety or high levels of stress have been observed to suffer from ulcers at higher rates and they get infected by H. pylori more often. Stress makes your immune system weaker and damages the digestive system, making it more susceptible to bacteria or microbes nearby. When you go through high stress, your body utilizes your energy to carry on other vital life functions apart from digesting the food properly and preventing the body from being infected by microbes. Natural stress relievers can help you manage stress better and the methods include regular mediation, exercise, and practice healing prayer, have fun outdoor, enough sleep and using essential oils to relieve from anxiety.

3. Boost immunity and control inflammation

Your immunity system can become weak by leading a highly inflammatory lifestyle and this will make your digestive system more prove to become infected with H. pylori bacteria. The bacteria itself can induce more inflammation inside the small intestine and the stomach, resulting in a malicious cycle that is difficult to break. Several researches show that nowadays around 30% to 40% of Americans suffer from H. pylori infection, although the infection remains dormant for years after years without any possible symptom.

H. pylori take part in ulcers by destroying the mucous coating that shields the wall of duodenum and the stomach from acids. Once this gets damaged, stomach acid get enter inside through the sensitive wall resulting in irritation and a burning sensation. The bacteria can spread through dirty water, utensils or food and also via body fluids, like the saliva. An ulcer will only occur if the person's immunity system is already weak due to other reasons. You can boost your immunity system to fight against infections by leaving poor lifestyle choices, such as drinking, smoking, imbalanced diet, processed food items, getting exposed to toxins, or an inactive lifestyle. These contribute to ulcer formation by weakening immunity and improving immunity. Some of these bad habits can also make it more difficult to treat your ulcers. Researchers have found out that smoking makes ulcers more difficult to heal and are more painful.

4. Eat low-processed, nutrient-rich food

An improper diet that contains less fresh fruits and vegetables and more packaged and processed foods, increases the risk of ulcers weakening immunity functions and enhancing inflammation. The ulcers symptoms are also worsen by skipping meals or eating only once or twice day or by eating a lot all at once. Therefore, it is rather the worst idea to skip breakfast. Eating spicy foods will also worsen the condition.

Foods that often cause gastric discomfort are caffeine, black pepper, red or hot chili pepper/powder, alcohol, peppermint, tomato products, coffee/tea, citrus juices and fruits, cola beverages, and fatty or fried foods. If you experience nausea or vomiting due to your ulcer, it is vital to take care of yourself in order to prevent dehydration, nutrient deficiencies and electrolyte imbalance. Patients with painful ulcers end up eating less to avoid the burning sensation or pain, however, by doing this they actually make the condition worse by consuming insufficient amount of nutrients and calories. If the consumed food lack in antioxidants, minerals and vitamins then the chance of getting deficiencies and inflammation increases greatly. Through food ulcers can be controlled by:

- Avoiding obesity and maintaining an adequate weight
- Don't eat stomach allergies or irritants food products
- Stop smoking and don't drink alcohol to save gut wall
- Eat frequently in small amounts throughout the day
- Stop eating 3 hours before bedtime
- Avoid consuming hot drinks and foods

❖ Ulcers that fail to heal

Refractory ulcers are peptic ulcers that cannot be healed with treatment. There are several reasons why ulcers fail to heal sometimes, and these are:

- Not following instructions while taking medicines
- Smoke tobacco regularly
- Certain types of H. pylori are resistant to antibiotics
- Use pain killers regularly, like aspirin, naproxen (Anaprox, Aleve, etc.) and ibuprofen (Motrin, Advil, etc.) as these increases the chance of getting ulcers.

Sometimes refractory ulcers are caused by:

- Stomach cancer
- Infections caused by other bacteria
- Disease, like Zollinger-Ellison syndrome, overproduces stomach acid
- Diseases, like Crohn's disease, causes ulcer-like sores in small intestine and stomach

Refractory ulcers are generally treated using different types of antibiotics to eliminate factors that prevent healing. You may need surgery if you are suffering from serious complications, like a perforation or acute bleeding. Nowadays, surgeries are needed rarely as many effective medicines are available now.

❖ Alternative medicine

Calcium carbonate containing medicines in over-the-counter pharmacies may help in treating peptic ulcers, although you should not use it as primary treatment option. Some evidences also shows that zinc can also help to heal ulcers. Ayurveda treatments to heal peptic ulcer include using turmeric, neem bark extract, mastic, cabbage, or deglycyrrhizinated licorice. These methods are not usually recommended as primary treatments as their effectiveness is not yet well known.

Prevention of Stomach Ulcers

In order to prevent the spread of H. pylori bacteria and decrease the chance of getting bacterial infection, wash your hands with water and soap properly and regularly. You must ensure to wash and cook your food properly. Ulcers caused by NSAIDs can be prevented by stopping or limiting the use of these drugs. If you must take these medicines, then follow the prescribed dosages strictly and don't drink alcohol. Some lifestyle changes can also prevent ulcers from occurring. These include limiting alcohol consumption, properly managing stress and avoiding tobacco products to keep your stomach wall healthy. In case of an emergency, call your doctor.

Chapter 4 – Recipes for Stomach Ulcer Patients

Unfortunately, gastric ulcer is a common disease of the GI tract. Several reports suggest that this illness occurs to 18% people among 1000. The advent of this illness is directly linked to our lifestyle and eating habits. Mucous tissue of your stomach goes through changes due to overeating/irregular eating, starvation, stress, drinking alcohol and smoking. Stomach ulcer patients can follow their treatment properly and prevent themselves from having relapse of the disease, by following a specific diet plan and eating only certain recipes. This chapter will not discuss about the general rules of nutrition and diet types, but instead will talk about different ways to enrich and diversify the menu with delicious recipes for the patients of stomach ulcer. Following a specific diet doesn't mean you have to cross out all the dishes from the menu that prompts your appetite. You can transform your everyday menu into something exotic by just adding some love and imagination. Some recipes are given below that stomach ulcer patients can enjoy.

1. **Milk Soup with Pumpkin**

Ingredients: 2 cups of water, 2 tablespoon of butter, 6 cups of milk, 4 teaspoon of sugar, 600 g of pumpkin, 4 tablespoon of semolina, and salt to taste.

Method: In the boiling milk, add the semolina and cook it for about 15 to 20 minutes. While this is cooking, cut the pumpkin into cubes and boil these in a little water. Smash the softened pumpkin along with the water to make broth. Pour the pumpkin smash in a pot and bring it to boil. Season the soup with some sugar and salt to taste.

2. Potato and Carrot Puree

Ingredients: 4 carrots, 8 to 10 potatoes, 2 cups of milk and 4 tablespoon of butter.

Method: At first peel the carrots and the potatoes and then boil them in hot water. While boiling, add salt to it. When softened, drain the broth and smash the veggies using a blender. Pour in warm milk, butter and then whip it.

3. Pate with Lean Meat

Ingredients: 2/3 of white loaf, parsley to taste 6 to 8 carrots, 2/3 cup of milk, 900 grams of lean meat of rabbit or veal, 400 g of chicken liver, 4 tablespoon of vegetable oil, 2 eggs, butter to taste and salt to taste.

Method: Cut the liver and the meat into small pieces, add water and boil these on low heat. Peel the carrots, cut these into chunks and add them to the boiling meat. Blend water and milk and soak the breads in this mixture. Mince the liver and meat and add the soaked bread without the crusts. Then mix together this meat mixture, eggs, parsley and salt.

Make small pate and cook them in the oven on oil-greased tray, for 40 to 45 minutes or until done.

4. Waist-Friendly Waldorf Salad

Traditionally, Waldorf salads are made with mayonnaise. This is not healthy to eat always. Exclude the mayo and you can eat a healthy recipe full of walnuts and fruits, rich in omega-3 fatty acids needed for superior brain function and a healthy heart.

Ingredients: ½ cup chopped walnuts, ¼ cup raisins, 1 tablespoon walnut oil, 2 large apples, cored and cubed and chopped 2 celery stalks, and ½ tablespoon apple cider vinegar, salt and pepper to taste.

Method: mix together the celery, apples, raisins and walnuts. In a separate bowl, whisk together the apple cider vinegar, walnut oil and the seasonings. Add this spice mixture to the salad, mix this well and serve on a bed of greens.

5. Sautéed Mackerel

Mackerel is one of the most fresh, wild fish that you can buy at a very reasonable price. This fish has a meaty texture and is full of mouth-watering flavor. Not only that, this fish is also rich in omega-3s.

Ingredients: 4 tablespoons olive oil, 4 (1/2 pound) mackerel fillets, lemon juice, salt and pepper to taste.

Method: On high flames, heat a sauté pan and pour in olive oil. Season the fish fillet and cook them in the hot pan. Sear them for 4 to 5 minutes. Flip and cook both the sides until they become golden brown on the outside but have a flaky white texture at the center. Squeeze a lemon over the top while serving.

Diet Plan for Stomach Ulcer Patients

Recently, many people believe that gastric ulcer and 12 duodenal ulcers can be easily treated using medicines to eradicate the bacteria H. pylori. The researchers have found that the microorganism is the main culprit behind the spreading of the illness in the body. The GI tract and the stomach will not recover very quickly as the healthy food did not completely lost their effectiveness. Doctors still advise patients to eat diet based on the nutritional values for these illnesses, particularly if they are leaking a lot for a long period of time. In this situation, the main harmful factor is the hydrochloric acid. For this you should eliminate products that increase the secretion of gastric juice.

You should pay attention to the food consistency. Pureed foods will not harm the stomach lining that much. The food that affect the mucosa mechanically are left out, only keeping the dishes in the menu that does not irritate and can be recycled. Patients must also reduce the amount of food consumption that is packed in flour coarse, coarse connective tissue meat or fiber. The functions of the stomach can be quickly restored by having dietetic food and therapeutic interventions. Patients are recommended to eat for 5 to 6 times per day. This is known as fractional power intake which refers to the most useful for all healthy and ill people. Too cold or too hot food should be avoided as these may harm more. All foods should be eaten at room temperature or lukewarm.

What Foods Can Be Eaten?

The diet for ulcer patients should be the medical diet that is prescribed for that patient to avoid heavy impact on the secretion. The simplest way to prepare food in this case is to use steam or grind in a blender. As for pastry, try to keep the white bread for the day before and the gallstone biscuits, dry biscuits and sweets for special occasions. Meat should be well cooked and the fish should be fresh. The patients should eat variety of dairy products, like milk and cheese, scrambled, boiled or cooked eggs. You should also eat different types of cereals (oatmeal, rice, semolina), made in a soft porridge soups, veggie soups or puddings and root vegetables.

You don't to eliminate vegetable oils and animal fats. You can add olive oil, sunflower oil, and butter in your foods in small amounts. In beverages, you can drink non-carbonated black tea and green compote of dried or fresh fruits in broth.

What Foods Cannot Be Eaten?

Ulcers patients need to exclude or limit the intake of foods that strongly stimulate the secretion. These include, soda, alcoholic beverages, coffee, strong tea and foods with preservatives and dyes. Foods that worsen your condition are fries, pickled, smoky and spicy dishes. Try to avoid these.

Too much fatty foods and canned foods can have adverse effect on the stomach. Limit the use of black bread and fresh hot white, fried peas, or fatty cream-filled pastries. You also need to eliminate ice cream, lard, mutton tallow, mushrooms and salt.

Recommended Servings of Food for Ulcer Patients

- **Menu for no pain/nausea or other symptoms in patients**

Stomach ulcer patients can follow the diet plan mentioned below for 2 days. Servings can be increased or decreased depending on the health of the person.

Day 1

✓ **Breakfast:** Start your day eating 2 soft-boiled eggs, 1 slice of bread and fruit jelly. Complimentary breakfast should be richer in nutrients, like white bread with buckwheat porridge and warm unsweetened tea.

✓ **Lunch and afternoon tea:** for this, take the first hash, the second boiled fish about a 100 g and then have them with boiled potatoes, white bread and stewed fruit. After 2 to 3 hours, eat 1 sandwich, 100g yogurt, butter and 1 peach.

✓ **Dinner:** eat veggie stew or boiled beef with braised cabbage, a glass of milk, fruit soufflé, figs or other fruits.

Day 2

- ✓ **Breakfast:** Eat 2 boiled eggs, jelly and white bread. After 2 hours, eat beef burgers, rice porridge with milk coffee.
- ✓ **Lunch and afternoon tea:** You can have milk or vermicelli soup with milk, mashed potato patties with warm and steamy sweet tea. After 3 hours, have dried apricots soaked in water or steamed, a glass of fruit jelly and a whole bread sandwich with butter and cheese and.
- ✓ **Dinner:** You should eat white bread, fish with steamed rice porridge. For dessert, have milk and apricot.

- **Menu served in severe pain after surgery**

Day 1

- ✓ **Breakfast:** Eat yogurt, bread and butter and water. After 2 hours, eat 2 soft-boiled eggs, mashed fruits, rice porridge and warm milk.
- ✓ **Lunch and afternoon tea:** You can have chicken soup with veggies, milk, and cooked pasta. For dessert, eat apple sauce and soaked apricots. After 3 hours, eat steam cutlets, mashed potatoes, soft white bread, raisins and broth hips.
- ✓ **Dinner:** Eat boiled beef with chopped veggies, salad of boiled root vegetables, fruit jelly and a glass of warm milk.

Day 2

✓ **Breakfast:** Start your day by eating healthy that includes mineral water, bread and butter. After 2 hours, eat semolina, sweet tea and steamed omelet.

✓ **Lunch and afternoon tea:** Make your menu exciting by including veggie soup with beef meatballs, boiled potatoes with their skins on and green peas and tea. After 3 hours, eat oatmeal, a slice of bread and milk.

✓ **Dinner:** You can eat veggie soup with, boiled boneless fish, milk, bread and boiled egg.

- **Useful tips and reviews**

Unhealthy lifestyle may encourage duodenal ulcer or stomach ulcer in relation with alcohol, stress, malnutrition and cigarettes. Most of the time, mental pressure or nervousness or tension can result in loss of appetite. On top of that, if you have a family medical history of stomach ulcer, you must be very careful concerning your health. If you are already suffering from peptic or stomach ulcer, you must strictly follow recommended diet.

As a natural treatment method, folk healers always advise to drink cabbage juice at least for 1 month. This remedy is very cheap and you must ignore its benefits. Instead of drinking tea or water, it is best for you to drink a solution made by mixing 1 tablespoon of honey in 1 glass of boiling water.

If your ulcer is caused due to smoking, you don't have any way other than leaving this bad habit. You can help yourself out by calming your nerves or think about something else to shift your focus away from cigarette.

In most cases, smoking is the best mode to develop an ulcer. Nicotine affects the central nervous system deeply by encouraging stimulation to the GI tract and the stomach. This chemical enters into the lungs while smoking and reaches the stomach via the saliva and inflames the mucosa. Ulcers don't heal easily and they continue to inflame. Around 5 times more smokers die from smoking ulcer than non-smokers and about 13% smokers develop tumors from their ulcers. Smoking tobacco enhances the secretion of mucous and causes heartburn. The liver is stimulated to wash the stomach by throwing a lot of bile. Toxins enter through the bile and duodenums and leave out hazardous untreated matters.

Conclusion

The effects of stomach ulcer are real and tangible and affect many of all around us. In order to feel better you just have to use some of the day-to-day techniques and implement certain mentioned diets into breakfast, lunch and dinner and do some useful lifestyle changes. You don't need to be as systematic as a computer or as punctual as a clock, trying is the first step and is the one that really matters. If you don't give it a shot how will you know if it works or not? You may find it hard to at first to change your habits but healthy living will keep you away from suffering due to stomach ulcer and give you relief if you already have the disease. The small steps may seem inconsequential but they go the distance to help alleviate your tummy ache. Soon your complications will neutralize, your body will work like a well-oiled machine, and heartburn with tummy ache will be a thing of the past.

Thank You for choosing this book! If you liked it, please take the time to share your experience on Amazon.com and rate the book. Thanks!

Printed in Great Britain
by Amazon